Guerrilla Apologetics
for
Life Issues

by Paul E. Nowak

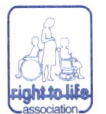

K-W and Area RTL Assoc.
215 Lancaster St. West
Kitchener, ON N2H 4T9
Phone/Fax: (519) 746-5433

Copyright © 2005 by Paul E. Nowak
All rights reserved. No part of this book may be reproduced or transmitted in any form or by any means, electronic or mechanical, including photocopying, recording, electronic file distribution, without permission in writing from the author.

Cover Photo: "Camo Series – Marine" Copyright © 2004 Andrew Ramsay. Used with Permission.
Cover Photo (Unborn Child at 20 weeks): Copyright © 2001 Life Issues Institute. Used with Permission.

Political Cartoons © 2002-2005 Paul A. Nowak. Initially published on CNSnews.com. Used with Permission.

ISBN 0-9772234-1-8

Special thanks to Steven Ertelt, who has been an example of dedication in putting women and children first.

Table of Contents

Introduction 1
Guerrilla Apologetics 101 7
Introduction to Logical Fallacies 13

When does life begin? 17

Can choices be wrong? 21

Is what is legal always right? 25

Does changing the words change the meaning? 27

Where is the proof of the masses lost to
unsafe, illegal abortions? 29

Is abortion safe? 33

Pro-abortion organizations: Non-profit or Industry? 39

What did the leaders of the early feminist
movement think about abortion? 49

Is population control a reason to justify abortion? 57

Where is the benefit of embryonic stem cell research? ..61

How is ending someone's life prematurely showing
respect for the elderly and disabled? 63

Is the death penalty really a deterrent to crime? 67

What if you're wrong? 71

Recommended Resources 74

Introduction

Since you have ventured to open this book, it can be reasonably assumed you consider yourself pro-life, or at least have an interest in the debate surrounding abortion, euthanasia, and other human life issues.

It can also be reasonably assumed that you have been asked, at least once, about your position on one or more of these issues. Recent years have brought discussions of scientific progress and ethics regarding human life to the forefront of political and social circles.

Some of you may rush headlong into discussions where you can express your views. Others may have strong convictions, but be unsure of how to communicate them with those who do not share your beliefs. Still others among you may be unsure of where you stand in the debate, but have not been able to avoid the discussions we all encounter in school, in the workplace, or even with family and friends in social settings.

The debate over life issues often comes up at inopportune times, or in places where it is culturally taboo to discuss them, such as in the workplace. At these times we do not have ready access to the wealth of information that has been published on the matter, and it is difficult for many of us to recall the volumes of information that could support our position. Time is usually limited as well, requiring us to come up with a short explanation that will also be effective in stating our position and helping the other person understand our view – and perhaps consider changing their own position.

This book's purpose is to be a tool for learning how to define and explain the pro-life position, while taking into consideration that we live in the "real world" with all its distractions and day-to-day activity.

While apologetics is usually a defense of one's religious beliefs, its broader definition includes the defense of any belief or position. This book instructs readers on the apologetics of the pro-life position, or a defense of the belief that human life should be protected at all stages from the moment of conception.

However, to stand only on the defensive is an ineffective tactic for discussing your position. In his *Art of War*, Sun Tzu even went so far as to say standing on the defensive indicated a weak position. At times, taking the defensive is perfectly fine, but it relies too heavily on knowing all the answers to the nearly infinite number of questions that might be posed.

It is never a good strategy in any competition (for such discussions are, in the spirit of good debate, competitions) to wear your opponent out by standing on the defensive. Boxers do not stand and block until their opponent collapses. Chess players know that if they only react to their opponent's moves, they will be less likely to win. Competitive sports cannot generally be won without scoring a few points during the struggle. Likewise, it is a very difficult (not to mention long) process to convince someone that your position is correct by waiting until you have convincingly answered all of his or her objections.

The method taught by this book is called "guerrilla," because the term refers to irregular warfare, and this book teaches "irregular" tactics for discussion and debate of life issues. The term has been adopted by the popular "Guerrilla Marketing" system, which emphasized the use of "irregular" tactics in marketing ideas or products, relying on strategy and not money to achieve maximum results.

The arguments and presentation of this book are "irregular," even for apologetics. Rather than simply stating facts and opinions, it relies on targeted questions intended to shake the foundations of someone arguing for the opposing position. Guerrilla tactics are not defensive, but offensive maneuvers.

Using a series of questions to argue a point has been a device employed since the time of Socrates. It has the advantage of being better received by someone who disagrees with you, while gently leading them to understand your argument. Given the need for pro-life arguments to be made quick and effective, it is an ideal method to employ in the life issues debate.

Because the arguments are disguised as questions, are meant to be used during day-to-day activities in our busy lives, and can be used to make short, targeted "attacks" on the beliefs of those that challenge pro-life advocates, the term "guerrilla" seems to adequately describe the method employed by this book.

Despite the reputation of the word "guerrilla," this book is intended to show you how to charitably take the offense in a discussion, while still targeting weak points in the opposition's logic. It should not be used in a way that will offend others with whom you are discussing the issue. No two people have had the same exact life experiences, or view things the same way. Sensitivity and understanding of the growth of others should be your utmost concern. Personally, I have experienced the most comfortable and mutually beneficial apologetics discussions by engaging in question-and-answer dialog with friends and acquaintances – sometimes lasting for hours.

In a nutshell, Guerrilla Apologetics is practiced in the flowing manner: When a discussion on an issue, in this case abortion, comes up, question the other person's position and allow them to question yours. Politely, calmly, and with an air of curiosity, ask questions from this book. Then allow them a chance to respond, and ask another question of you.

In this way you can set up and maintain a dialog in which to argue the issue, instead of a quarrel. Always refrain from making personal attacks or criticizing another's beliefs, even if they are overly critical of yours. Avoid hostile discussions, and walk away if the discussion is deteriorating into a shouting match. Your goal should be to plant seeds of knowledge that have the potential to change their position – you cannot change their mind, they must convince themselves. Do not let pride drive you to try to prove them wrong by the end of the conversation, or change their position on the spot. If you fail to exercise tact and civility, your actions and tone will overshadow and taint your efforts.

Cartoon by Paul Nowak, originally published by CNSnews.com on 10/18/02

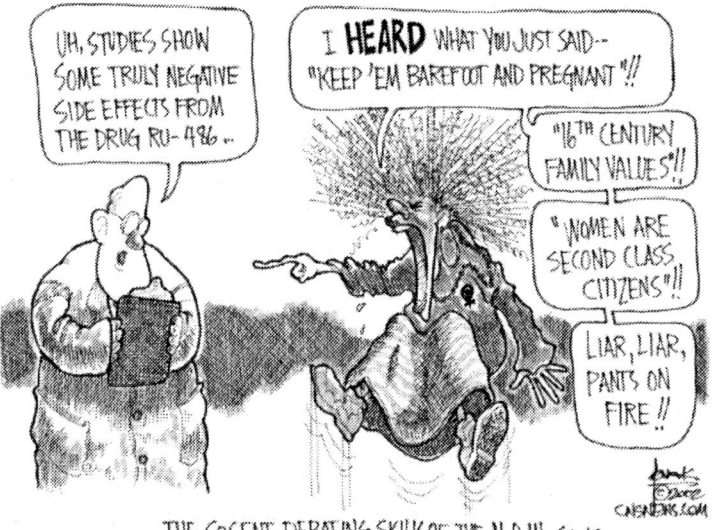

If the "discussion" degenerates to this level, it is probably best to walk away.

Most importantly, keep your friendship intact – if the discussion becomes too heated with a friend, take some time away from the subject.

Phrase your questions carefully – the ones listed in this book are an example. Do not accuse, as in "Why do you approve of the murder of children?" but instead, ask a question about their position and why they believe it. (Example, "When do you believe human life begins, and why?")

On a final note, this book is not written from any particular religious position, as the supporters and opponents of abortion profess a wide range of faiths. In order to gather the widest possible support for the cause for life, and as there are so many logical and common-sense reasons to support it, the questions and arguments are written to appeal to the common logic and morality of all humanity, not those of a particular faith. This approach has the added advantage of not alienating an opponent by assuming they hold a religious belief or spiritual writing in the same regard that you do. It also makes the arguments themselves stronger by virtue of their own merit as true facts, and impervious to claims that they are motivated by one's personal beliefs.

In Defense of Life,

Paul E. Nowak

Guerrilla Apologetics 101

Before going into the details of using Guerrilla Apologetics, it is important that the goal is made clear. The purpose of using Guerrilla Apologetics is to turn the discussion into a conversation with give-and-take on both sides.

You should NOT try to prove the other person wrong, or change their position on the spot. Your arguments, no matter how good they are, cannot change someone else's mind. Only they can do that – it is important that they choose to change their mind. While your arguments and questions, and especially your openness to discuss life issues may play a large role in their decision, much of the time we do not see the immediate effects of the part we play.

Remember, your goal is to set up and maintain a discussion, not a shouting match. To keep tempers from flaring, refrain from making personal attacks or criticizing another's beliefs, even if they are overly critical of yours.

Attitude is everything in Guerrilla Apologetics. If you fail to exercise tact and civility, your actions and tone will overshadow and taint your efforts. Ask questions with sincere curiosity, and respect the other person as an expert on what they believe is true. After all, you would be offended if someone stereotyped you based on your position, and accused you of not knowing what you were talking about. Therefore do not make that same assumption about them. Your sensitivity and understanding to others' beliefs will often lead them to exercise similar sensitivity and understanding to yours. Remember, they believe their position to be right at least as strongly as you believe that your position is correct.

Most importantly, keep your friendship intact – if the discussion becomes too heated with a friend, take some time away from the subject.

The following conversation illustrates the Guerrilla Apologetics method:

Let's assume that in the usual course of business at school, at work, or around the neighborhood someone approaches you and asks, "You're pro-life, right? Why do you think ..."

Answer their question to the best of your ability. Use factual information as much as possible, but not all of us can keep so much information mentally accessible. Take a deep breath, and consider your answer before you say it. Think your answer through; terminology is everything and a slip of the tongue can make your message more difficult to understand.

If you don't have the answer ready, or honestly don't know, go ahead and admit it. Let the other person know that you'll look into it and get back to them. When you get a chance use one or more of the resources found at the end of this book to find the answer. You can say something like, "That's a good question, but I don't have the answer now. I'll make sure I can get a proper explanation for you later."

If you do have an answer, keep it as brief as possible. Give them the reason you believe what you do. Sometimes the question will be a misunderstanding that you will have to clear up. Do so courteously; while the other person may not have understood what they were asking about, no one likes to be told they are wrong, or for a big deal to be made out of their ignorance.

Once you have made a response, either a refutation, clarification, or a promise to find an answer for them, proceed to ask them a question. Lead in with something like:

"While we're discussing what we think about abortion (or the issue at hand), what do you think about..."

How you ask this first question is important; especially since your challenger may not be prepared for you to inquire about *their* beliefs.

Do not interrupt them if they start to ask another question immediately after you respond to their first question, let them finish and then ask if you can ask a question before answering their second one.

Also, do not presume to know what you are talking about regarding what they believe – there are a great many reasons for people to hold beliefs and positions different from yours, and some may come from personal experiences that have left very strong perceptions. So do not accuse them in your question – ask, "When do you believe life begins?" instead of, "Why do you think mothers should be allowed to kill their children?"

Keep in mind the discussion is only going to progress if you discuss the issue on common ground. The two questions above are good examples of this principle – the first assumes only that the other person believes life begins at some point (a very reasonable assumption unless the person believes people never do have life). The second question presupposes that the other person believes the unborn child is alive, and impugns that they approve of mothers killing their children, such as in the case of Andrea Yates and Susan Smith. The first question seeks to challenge and understand more of what the other person believes, the second is a prejudiced question that assumes the other person approves of crimes considered reprehensible by most people. The second question will be a turn-off, and after you have offended the person you will not be able to discuss the issue openly.

Remember that you cannot criticize another's position unless you both acknowledge a common idea. For instance, abortion cannot be murder in the mind of someone who does not believe that the unborn child is a living person. Thus you cannot accuse them of supporting murder. However, if the person believes that the unborn person is alive in the last three months of pregnancy, there is common ground (during that last trimester) where you might point out to them that ending the life of a living person is murder. Since they agree with you that the unborn child at that point is living human being, you can use reason to argue that abortion is murder in that case.

For this very reason you should try as much as possible to keep religion out of the discussion, unless you share the same religious beliefs as the other person. For instance, if you are Catholic and are discussing the issue with another Catholic, you very well can (and in my opinion, should!) cite the common faith's unwavering pro-life position. If you are a Christian discussing with another Christian, your churches may not teach the same social morality on life issues, but you may use commonly held elements of the faith, such as the command to be "fruitful and multiply" in Genesis, or any biblical passage that extols the virtues of having children (rather than avoiding ways to have them, such as abortion), or Christ's prophecy that has apparently come to pass:

> Jesus turned and said to them, "Daughters of Jerusalem, do not weep for me; weep for yourselves and for your children. For the time will come when you will say, 'Blessed are the barren women, the wombs that never bore and the breasts that never nursed!' Then they will say to the mountains, 'Fall on us!' and to the hills, 'Cover us!' For if men do these things when the tree is green, what will happen when it is dry?"
> (Luke 23:28-31 NIV)

The questions given in each section of this book are worded to be open-ended, so feel free to use them as a guide in formulating questions to ask. Following each question is further background for reference – including factual information, including statistics and news stories, that support the underlying pro-life position.

Once you have asked a question, give your challenger time to respond. Again, they may be surprised that you have challenged them, and they may not be familiar with the subject matter you have brought up. If the pause gets rather long and awkward, or they seem lost, give them a way out by saying, "If you're not sure, that's O.K., I was just curious.

Did you have another question for me?" If they had asked a second question, remind them of it so they can resume the conversation easily. A question that stumps them may have great impact, but if you relieve their awkwardness kindly, your attitude will make them more open to sharing their position with you and more receptive to your contributions.

While you will be challenging them to re-examine their position, which they may find uncomfortable, do your best to make them feel comfortable in discussing what they believe, and asking you about yours. Do your best to alternate asking questions and responding to questions, and always maintain a sense of calm, even if your challenger gets emotional.

If you happen to get into a debate with someone who you can not maintain a conversation with, such as someone who incessantly lectures you, criticizes your beliefs repeatedly, or simply will not give you a chance to get a word in edgewise, excuse yourself and try to get some distance from them, at least for the moment. Not everyone will be receptive to an open discussion, and there is no point to tying to speak with someone who will not listen. Perhaps at some other time they will be more open to a conversation about their position on life issues.

Again, remember that a personal relationship, even with co-workers, acquaintances, and enemies, is far more important than winning a debate. The manner in which you conduct yourself and treat others is far more powerful than any argument, however witty and true it is.

An Introduction to Logical Fallacies

Truth generally has a way of coming out in the end. However, we as human beings are not purely reasoning creatures, and our personal experiences and beliefs taint our arguments and decisions.

Since, unlike *Guerrilla Apologetics for Catholics*, the issues discussed in this book are based on truth and falsehood, and not faith and beliefs, there is a great deal more rational thinking and logic needed to effectively discuss the issues.

Most importantly, a pro-life advocate who is or expects to enter into discussions with people who hold the opposing position must be aware of the dominant logical fallacies – not only to recognize them when they are used by your opponent, but so that you can avoid using them yourself.

The first is called the **Straw Man**. This fallacy involves attacking an argument that the other person never made. For example: you argue that RU-486 has caused a number of deaths and the safety of the drug is in question. Your opponent says that a Dark Ages philosophy of women's rights has no place in the 21st century. Rather than address the argument you made, your opponent has torn down a "Straw Man" (often at considerable length) to give the appearance of a stronger counter-argument, although it has nothing or little to do with the original statement you made.

You can counter the Straw Man by revisiting the original statement, for instance: "I agree that women have been treated unfairly in the past, and we should not return to such practices, but I do not see how questioning the safety of a drug that has caused women's deaths is related to treating women unfairly."

You might even use their "straw" argument to press the original argument, although this depends on the arguments you both have made. For example: "Actually, doesn't the idea of an unsafe drug, exclusively made for women, being put on the market constitute an unfair practice against women?"

Another common fallacy is **Hasty Generalization**, in which a general argument is made on a small sample of information. For instance, if one says: "The teens I asked are sexually active, so therefore all teens, including yours, must be also." This is countered by pointing out a more representative sample, or by showing that one cannot use such a small sample to draw such a general conclusion. (An example that uses the same logical fallacy but would probably be considered absurd is that all American soldiers must be sexual deviants because of the handful involved in the sexual humiliation of Iraqi prisoners.)

Fallacy of Exclusion is difficult to detect, but it is common. When someone makes an argument but leaves out a particular fact that would contradict the conclusion, they commit the Fallacy of Exclusion. This was committed on a grand scale by a 2004 Oxford study on the abortion-breast cancer link. Considered by many pro-abortion groups as the "end-all" study on the matter, it consisted of a comprehensive review of over 50 studies on the possible link of abortion to breast cancer. While the conclusion was that no such link existed, the study's lead author, Valarie Beral, admitted to the *Washington Post* that they excluded many studies that *had* found a link and contradicted their conclusion, citing only an unproven belief that women with breast cancer "are more likely than healthy women to reveal they had an abortion, leading to the conclusion that there are more abortions among this group." The failure to include data that compromised the desired conclusion is evidence of a Fallacy of Exclusion.

While difficult to detect unless you know the facts that have been excluded, the Fallacy of Exclusion can be countered by pointing out the information that was excluded.

In the case of a **Post Hoc** fallacy, an argument is made that because something happened before a certain result, the preceding action was the cause. When a certain region experiences a decline in teen abortions, Planned Parenthood usually claims that their efforts are the reason, despite the fact that they encourage sexual activity in teenagers, are the nation's largest abortion provider, and recommend abortion over adoption in most cases. To counter this fallacy, point out other circumstances that may have caused the result. The counter argument is strengthened if there is evidence that the other factors have been shown to be effective in other cases.

In the example used above, abstinence programs and parental notification laws have been shown to be effective in many states where they have been put into practice. The repeatability of these results, compared to the efforts of Planned Parenthood across the country (where the number of abortions are rising in some areas and decreasing in others, despite the use of similar programs nationwide), shows that the parental notification and abstinence programs have a greater likelihood of being the real cause for the decline.

This is meant only to be a brief summary of a just handful of logical fallacies you may encounter. For more information on fallacies, consult a legal education resource. "Stephen's Guide to the Logical Fallacies" (http://www.datanation.com/fallacies/) is a terrific Internet resource on the subject.

Question 1: When does life begin?

This is a simple question, yet it quite often goes unanswered by those who advocate abortion. When exactly does one's "right to life" begin?

The argument that an unborn child is only a "potential" human life is often made, but an explanation of when the child actually becomes a human life worthy of protection is not addressed. The lack of a definition, or even consideration, of when life begins opens the door to numerous other abuses of life, and is therefore an important question.

Also, consider that one of the most trusted forms of forensic evidence is DNA testing. Each person's DNA makeup is their own, identifying the individual and distinguishing them from every other human being on the planet.

That DNA is stored in chromosomes in every cell of the body. Each species has a number of chromosomes that is typical for its kind. In the case of humans, the normal number is 23 pairs, or 46 total chromosomes. With too many or too few chromosomes, abnormalities occur, leading to death or developmental problems.

A human being's identity is therefore established at the moment of conception when the sperm and the ovum, each with 23 chromosomes, unite to form a new organism with 46 chromosomes. Once combined, the chromosomes line up and the individual's DNA is set – every single cell of that individual human is formed from that initial union, and will contain the same unique DNA code.

Why is this considered to be the moment of life's beginning?

First, after conception, the cell begins to replicate and the embryo grows. No need to consult scientists on this, ask any kindergarten student why a tree is alive and a rock is not. They will tell you the tree grows and is therefore alive. A slightly more advanced student will also tell you the living organism needs nutrients, but of course that is not contested by pro-abortion advocates who argue that the mother sustains the "growth" within her and therefore has a right to do as she wishes with it.

The second reason conception is the moment of life's beginning is the fact that the growing organism within the mother is an individual human life. It is a new, living, growing embryo whose DNA does not match that of its father, or even its mother who carries it.

The unborn child's blood never mixes with its mother's, and yet oxygenated blood flows through it. Nutrients are passed from the mother's blood to the baby through the placenta, just as oxygen and nutrients pass from the lungs to the blood and from the blood to organs in an adult body. Each and every cell of the child's, including the blood, contains that unique DNA that will never alter or change. In fact, because of the separation of the mother and child, an HIV-positive mother will not usually pass the disease onto her child while it is inside of her – the greatest risk of infection comes during delivery.

Such facts disarm several pro-abortion arguments, such as

the statement that the child is part of the mother's body for her to do with as she pleases (like her hair or her fingernails that she is entitled to cut off). But the truth is, *her* hair and nails contain *her* DNA, and are part of *her* body, while her baby does not have her DNA, and is not actually part of her body.

But is the organism within her a parasite, like a "worm" or "bug" to be removed? No, as it has the genetic identification of a human being – 46 chromosomes, separating it from the species of parasitic organisms, and requiring the classification of "human."

Defining any other point as the beginning of life is variable. The heart begins beating at about three weeks, and the baby can survive outside of the mother's womb after about seven months (even earlier in many cases), and of course birth seldom occurs exactly when predicted. Like any other milestone in human development, such as the ability to walk, to talk, or the onset of puberty or age-related disabilities, the development in the womb occurs at a different pace for each individual, and defies labeling an age or developmental stage as the moment of life's beginning.

If a variable stage were to be defined as the moment of life's beginning, what would prevent the moving of the line to allow for the termination of life a few minutes, hours, or days after birth, or based upon one's dependence on parental care for shelter and nourishment? (Especially when that stage that can sometimes last until adulthood.)

Ask your opponent, when do they believe life begins? If they say birth, ask them about 1 minute before, 1 hour before, 1 day before, 1 month before. See if you can get them to define a moment of life's beginning in which abortion would be acceptable. Ask them where their scientific reasoning is for their "belief" - and see who really is arguing about their beliefs and who is arguing based on scientific fact.

A great many pro-abortionists believe after 3 months of pregnancy the baby is "alive." Ask them about the day before. What great change takes place exactly three months after conception? Keep asking questions and it will become evident that no exact moment in pregnancy, except conception, can be defined as the moment of life's beginning.

As this question is almost never asked, considered, or brought up in pro-abortion materials, it is a powerful question (or series of questions) to ask another when discussing the right to life.

Question 2: Can Choices be Wrong?

Those who support abortion refer to their position as "pro-choice." While polling data shows that many people identify themselves under this title, it is grossly misleading.

Choice is not a right, it is a responsibility. It cannot be taken from you, in fact it is more inseparable than your own life. For example, when faced with certain death one can choose to die bravely or struggle, to mourn or to plead; your life can be taken but choice cannot.

Choice of itself cannot be made "legal" or "moral," because choice is necessary to perform an action that is legal or illegal, moral, or immoral. It is the ability choose that makes us saints or monsters. It is what gives us ability and accountability; it is the glory and burden of being human.

Every human atrocity began with a human choice. To advocate choice is to advocate and approve of every choice in the Pandora's Box of human ability, compassionate or destructive, from self-sacrifice to the atom bomb.

In fact, if you were to review human history, you would find bad human choices behind every war, every tragedy, and every act of terrorism that reveals the inhumanity of humans.

To be "pro-choice" is to be in support of an ability to choose, but the ability to choose is never truly endangered, and is never right or correct in and of itself. Life, on the other hand, is frequently lost to the choices of others. Has a

Cartoon by Paul Nowak, originally published by CNSnews.com on 12/05/02

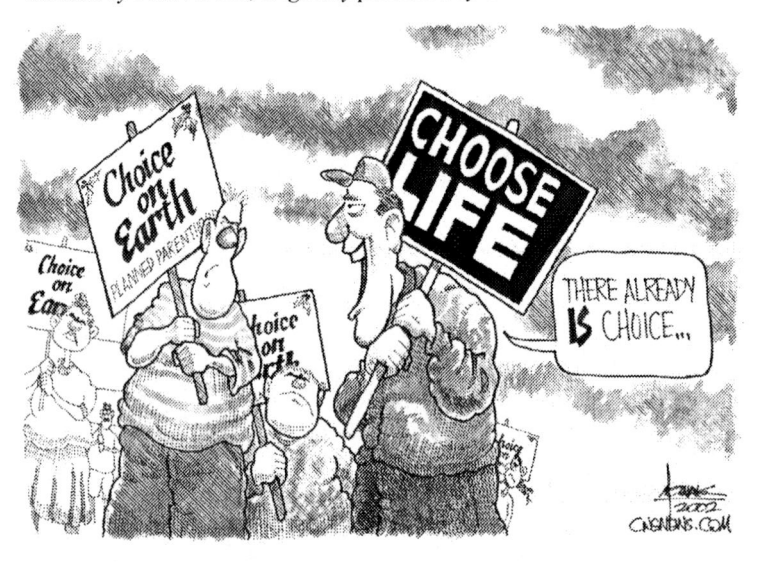

22

"pro-choice" activist yet stood up for a serial killer's "right to choose" his actions?

Advocates for another tragic assault on human freedoms also referred to themselves as supporters of the individual's right to choose. Public figures who advocated slavery in the 19th century did not adopt a "pro-slavery" stance, but rather a position approving of a slave owner's right to *choose* to hold slaves.

This "right to choose," or, as it is also known today, "pro-choice," position was held by Stephen Douglas, the presidential candidate who put forth the pro-choice position well during the Lincoln-Douglas debates:

> "The great principle is the right of everyone to judge and decide for himself, whether a thing is right or wrong, whether it would be good or evil for them to adopt it; and the right of free action, the right of free thought, the right of free judgment upon the question is dearer to every true American than any other under a free government. ... It is no answer to this argument to say that [it] is an evil and hence should not be tolerated. You must allow the people to decide for themselves."

What defense attorney in his right mind would ever try to use such logic to defend a murderer? Certainly a right to choose is not an unlimited right.

Douglas' opponent saw the glaring flaw in such logic, and responded during the debate: "No one has the right to do what is wrong."

Abraham Lincoln won the election, and is considered a national hero. Where is the memorial for the champion of choice, Stephen Douglas?

Question 3: Is what is legal always right?

The issue of slavery highlights another flaw in the logic of pro-abortion arguments. Does the legality of an act necessarily mean it is always right?

In 1857, the Supreme Court ruled 7-2 on *Dred Scott v. Sandford*, declaring that slaves were the lawful property of the owner. They had no standing as citizens, there were not the "people" referred to in "We the people," nor were they to be recognized as having "unalienable rights" of "life, liberty, and the pursuit of happiness."

Slavery was legal. And yet it is considered wrong today.

In 1973 the Supreme Court ruled 7-2 on *Roe v. Wade*, declaring that a woman had the "right to terminate her pregnancy." The language used in *Roe* is remarkably similar to the wording used in the *Dred Scott* decision, except that instead of referring to "negroes, " the Court states that "the unborn have never been recognized in the law as persons in the whole sense."

The point here is not that the Supreme Court is flawed, but merely that the august body is not infallible. It can be wrong. It can, and has, declared something that is wrong to be legal. To state it bluntly, what is legal is not always right.

The *Dred Scott* decision is only one example of a government's authorization of actions that have been universally denounced as wrong. It has been cited here because it was made by the the same governing body that made the *Roe* decision over 100 years later.

For instance, the United States was not the only country to declare slavery to be legal. Also, the imprisonment of citizens of Japanese descent during WWII could hardly be considered right, nor could what happened to the Jews in Germany and throughout Europe in the same period. However, within their respective governments, such atrocities were legal.

Question 4: Does changing the words change the reality?

Advocates of abortion often use different language than pro-life advocates. Abortion is a "termination of pregnancy," and the unborn child is a "product of a pregnancy" or more commonly, a "fetus."

But let's consider their use of language. For instance, a termination is the ending of something – like saying a landlord "terminated the lease" instead of saying they evicted you.

Merriam-Webster defines "Pregnant" as "containing unborn young within the body." Note that it does not say "containing tissue matter"or "containing potential life."

The same dictionary defines "abortion" as it relates to the medical procedure as "the termination of a pregnancy after, accompanied by, resulting in, or closely followed by the death of the embryo or fetus."

Fetus, now commonly used in English to refer to an unborn child, comes from the Latin word for "offspring." Putting it all together, abortion is the ending (termination) of the carrying of unborn young (pregnancy) when related to the death of one's offspring (fetus).

But how does this play into our discussion of when life begins? Well, if abortion is contingent on the death of the unborn being, then doesn't it assume that it was alive before?

To put it simply, how does something that is not alive die? Or how does something end that has not yet begun?

Abortion by its definition ends something. When related to pregnancy, it ends life.

Changing the words does not change the reality of what occurs.

Question 5: Where is the proof for the masses lost to unsafe, illegal abortions?

You probably have heard the argument that if abortion was illegal millions of women would have to resort to dangerous, back alley abortions and could die at the hands of unlicensed "back alley butchers," just as thousands of women died before abortion was legalized.

In response, ask them for their proof. After all, the burden of proof falls on the one making the argument.

Next, point out what other pro-abortion advocates have said when ultimately faced with the lack of proof for their claims.

Co-founder of NARAL (National Abortion Rights Action League), Dr. Bernard Nathanson stated in his book, *Aborting America*:

> "How many deaths were we talking about when abortion was illegal? In N.A.R.A.L. we generally emphasized the drama of the individual case, not the mass statistics, but when we spoke of the latter it was always '5,000 to 10,000 deaths a year.' **I confess that I knew the figures were totally false, and I suppose the others did too if they stopped to think of it**. But in the 'morality' of the revolution, it was a useful figure, widely accepted, so why go out of our way to correct it with honest statistics. The overriding concern was to get the laws

eliminated, and anything within reason which had to be done was permissible."
(Emphasis Added)

According to the U.S. Bureau of Vital Statistics, only 39 women died from illegal abortions in 1972, the year before legalization. If abortion was in such great demand and so dangerous, wouldn't the number of deaths be higher?

Here's another common-sense argument: If 10,000 women died each year from illegal abortions, wouldn't it be noticed? In 1970, there were 842,553 female deaths of all ages according to the Center for Disease Control. That would mean that more than one in every 100 female deaths, regardless of age, would have been from an abortion.

For comparison, in 2001 (a point in recent memory) .84 people per 100 died from homicide. That's less than the 1.18 toddler, school-age, teen, adult, and elderly women per 100 that would have died from illegal abortions in 1970, if the pro-abortion "statistics" were true. Wouldn't such an incredible rate have been well-documented and obvious?

But the low death rate was known and reported even before *Roe v. Wade*. Thirteen years before the legalization of abortion, Dr. Mary Calderon, medical director of Planned Parenthood, made the following admission in the July 1960 edition of the *American Journal of Public Health:*

> "90% of illegal abortions are being done by physicians. Call them what you will, abortionists, or anything else, they are still physicians, trained as such; ... They must do a pretty good job if the death rate is as low as it

is... Abortion, whether therapeutic or illegal, is in the main no longer dangerous, because it is being done well by physicians."

Today's largest national abortion provider admitted that illegal abortions were mostly performed by trained physicians, that there were few deaths, and that abortion, more than a decade before its legalization, was "no longer dangerous!"

If even Planned Parenthood admitted that abortions were safe prior to the legalization of abortion, and a co-founder of NARAL admitted the "thousands" of deaths they cited were a complete fabrication, where did pro-abortion advocates get those statistics?

Thin air. Dispute the statistics by asking for proof, and they will be unable to stand by that argument anymore.

Question 6: Is abortion safe?

Abortion advocates equate "legal abortion" with "safe abortion." Now that abortion is legal, is it really safe?

Keep in mind that the Alan Guttmacher Institute, the research arm of Planned Parenthood, found that only 5 percent of abortions were done for the mother's physical or psychological health. So abortion itself is seldom used for health purposes.

(On a brief side note, less than one percent of abortions are preformed for rape or incest, two other reasons often cited by pro-abortionists. However, just because the crime of rape was committed against the mother, it is not necessary to hand down a death sentence on the child.)

Dr. Daniel J. Martin, clinical instructor at St. Louis University Medical School summed up the effects of abortion well in his paper, "The Impact of Legal Abortion on Women's Minds and Bodies."

"The impact of abortion on the body of a woman who chooses abortion is great and always negative," he wrote in 1993. "I can think of no beneficial effect of a social abortion on a body."

Cartoon by Paul Nowak, originally published by CNSnews.com on 10/24/03

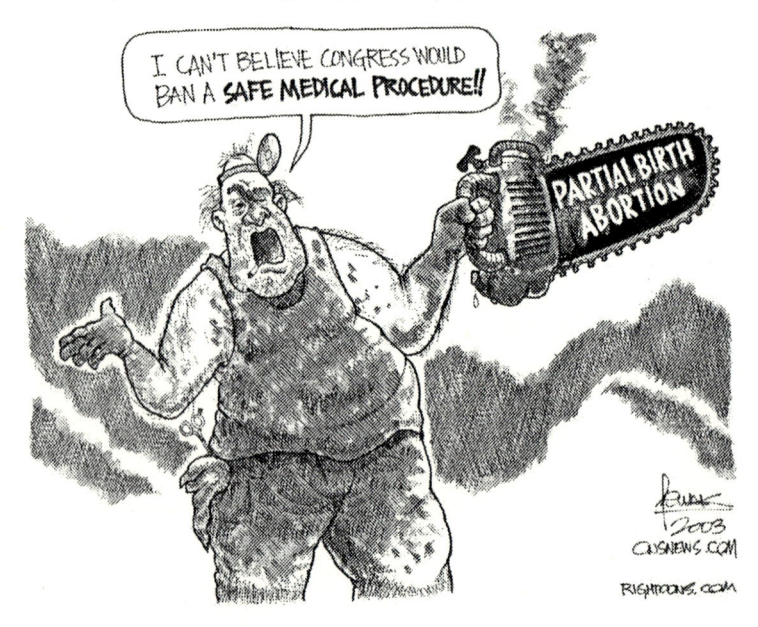

In 2003 a ban on partial birth abortions was signed into law. Opposition to this "safe" and "necessary" procedure was voiced, even though the procedure required the mother to undergo delivery of most of the child before it was killed, making it no safer, in fact even more dangerous, than giving birth.

Cartoon by Paul Nowak, originally published by CNSnews.com on 11/10/03

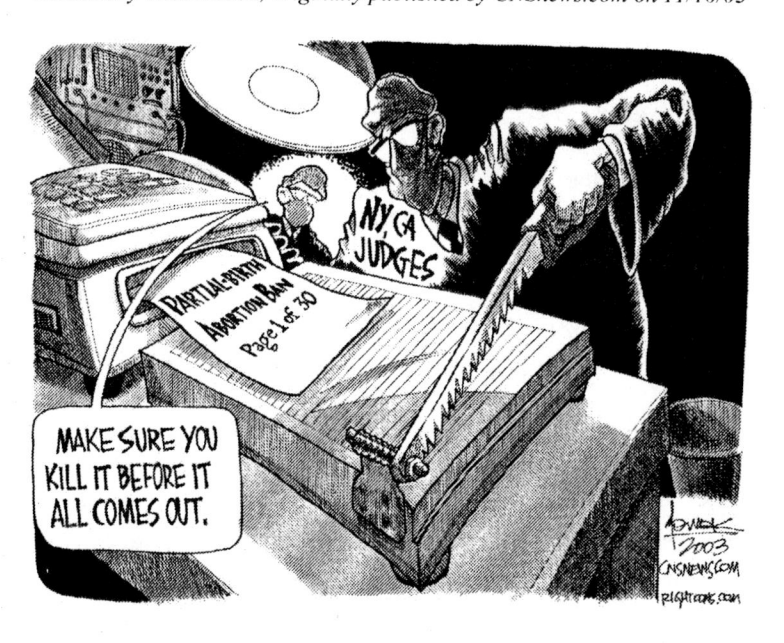

Ironically, the ban was blocked by judges in New York, California, and Nebraska immediately after it was signed into law. Pro-abortion groups filed lawsuits alleging the ban did not adequately protect the safety of the mother.

A great many statistics can be brought up here, but as this book is meant to serve as a quick guide, there is not enough room. For a compilation of statistics on post-abortion complications, there is no better source than the Elliot Institute, which publishes *Detrimental Effects of Abortion: An Annotated Bibliography with Commentary*, listed in the references section at the end of this booklet. It is an entire publication that consists only of references to studies that have scientifically shown that abortion is not safe.

Without statistics on hand, the way to address this question is to consider the procedures, which almost all involve inserting sharp objects into the woman. Does this not constitute a danger?

The truth is, women still die from abortion. Even something as "safe" as the abortion pill, which works by cutting off blood flow to the uterus, has been known to cause infections and excessive bleeding, as well as death.

Another growing concern is a link of abortion to breast cancer. As the baby grows within the mother, her breasts prepare to feed the baby. However, the cells that develop in her breasts during the pregnancy do not begin to turn into milk-producing cells until late in the pregnancy. If the pregnancy is stopped early, those cells remain, and have been shown in many studies to be more prone to cancer than cells allowed to mature. This risk factor is in addition to other, more widely accepted breast cancer risk factors associated with abortion, including childlessness, smaller family size, and doing little or no breastfeeding.

Cartoon by Paul Nowak, originally published by CNSnews.com on 4/19/02

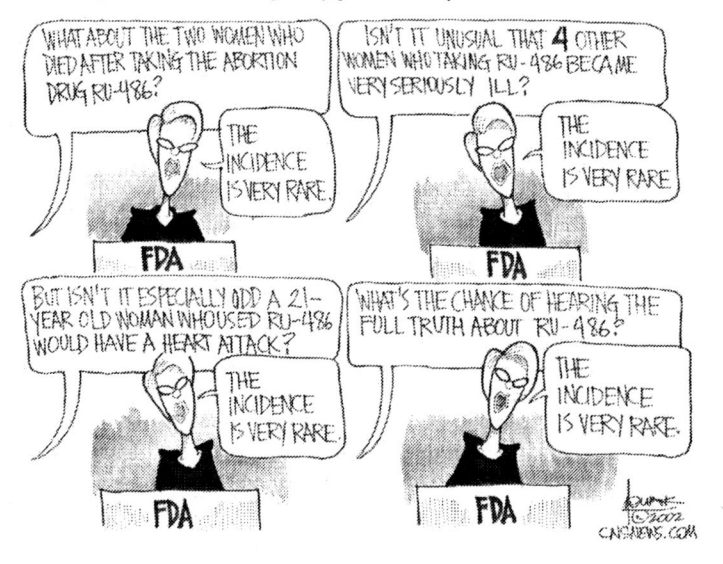

As for mental consequences, if postpartum depression is a documented fact after full term pregnancies, and depression is a recognized symptom following a miscarriage, how could there be no such side effect to an early and willed end to the pregnancy?

Arguing that abortion is unsafe can very well be like trying to argue with someone who thinks gravity pulls away from the earth. There's just too much scientific evidence that says otherwise. Ask questions to get your opponent really thinking about the "safety" of abortion, and when possible present them with some results from studies to provide the documented evidence. The website www.afterabortion.org is a good place to find such information quickly.

Question 7: Do pro-abortion organizations resemble non-profits, motivated by what is best for humanity, or other industries, motivated by money?

At first this might seem like an absurd question. Pro-abortion groups are almost all registered non-profits. However, Planned Parenthood, the most vocal pro-abortion organization, also happens to be the largest abortion provider in the United States. Its practices and financial data defies the common image of a non-profit, even though it claims such status.

STOPP International, part of the American Life League, has monitored the financial reports of Planned Parenthood since 1987. These reports are posted every year on Planned Parenthood's website and are public information.

Between July 1, 2002 and June 30, 2003, Planned Parenthood had an income of $766.6 million, a 10.7% increase over the previous year. It reported $688 million in net assets at the end of the year, and its revenues exceeded its expenses by $36.6 million – a larger "profit" than some corporations are able to report.

Hundreds of millions in revenue and assets, 10% growth and a "profit" every year since 1987 (maybe more, but STOPP began watching the reports closely since then) – Planned Parenthood would not be a bad investment, if it were not for the fact it is a registered non-profit.

Where does all that money come from? In the fiscal year ending in 2003 the largest share of that revenue came from clinic income, accounting for 36% ($288.2 million), government grants and contracts provided 33% ($254.4 million), and private contributions accounted for 30% ($228.1 million).

Abortion, STOPP estimates, accounted for approximately $90.9 million in revenue, based on Planned Parenthood reporting 227,375 abortions preformed between July 2002 and June 2003, and an average cost of $400 per abortion. Totaling the statistics from 1977-2003, STOPP has estimated that abortion has provided Planned Parenthood with $985 million in revenue. By the time you are reading this, the revenue has most likely exceeded $1 billion.

Even though Planned Parenthood lobbies for tax dollars and pleads for donations, it has more money than it can spend. And employees don't do badly either. Gloria Feldt, the organization's former President, was paid $363,426 in 2002-2003 fiscal year.

However, while Planned Parenthood is the nations largest abortion provider, its 190+ facilities only represent 17% of all abortion businesses. Abortion is a billion-dollar industry.

So why bring up this information? It will put some of Planned Parenthood's actions and positions into perspective.

While it says it promotes "choice," Planned Parenthood routinely opposes any measure that infringes on its interests – even if the measure is in the interest of the women it claims to serve.

Cartoon by Paul Nowak, originally published by CNSnews.com on 1/15/03

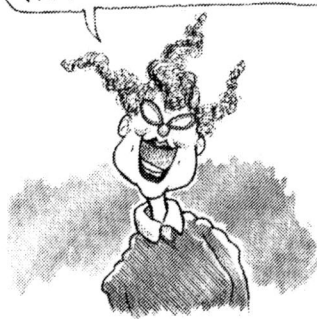

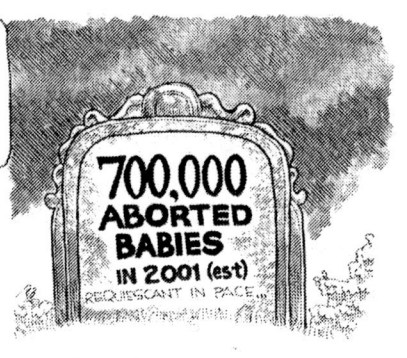

Planned Parenthood makes money from abortions, a fact that was demonstrated earlier, but they do not profit from other "options" they claim to offer women. For instance, Planned Parenthood is not in any way an adoption agency and thus must refer outside their organization for that.

According to Planned Parenthood's own reports, from 1997 to 2002 their adoptions referrals dropped by 79% (from 9,381 to 1,963), but abortions increased by 37.7%. In fact, in 2002 Planned Parenthood preformed 115 abortions for each adoption referral it made. It would appear that Planned Parenthood is far from impartial when giving women a choice of options.

Planned Parenthood opposes clinic regulations, despite the fact that in many states there are more restrictions on veterinary clinics than self-regulated abortion facilities. Such regulations, including requirements to be covered by malpractice insurance, would cut into the profit margin of the business – in fact, such laws have led to abortion businesses closing due to the increased financial costs.

They have also vehemently opposed legislation requiring women to wait 24 hours before an abortion and to receive information about the risks and alternatives.

Planned Parenthood opposes parental notification and consent laws, and even provides information on its site for teens to circumvent such laws where they exist by seeking a judicial waver. A woman's right to "choose" apparently ends when the "choice" becomes old enough to be sexually active herself.

Cartoon by Paul Nowak, originally published by CNSnews.com on 4/28/04

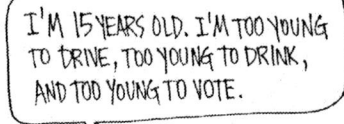

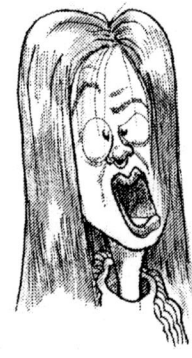

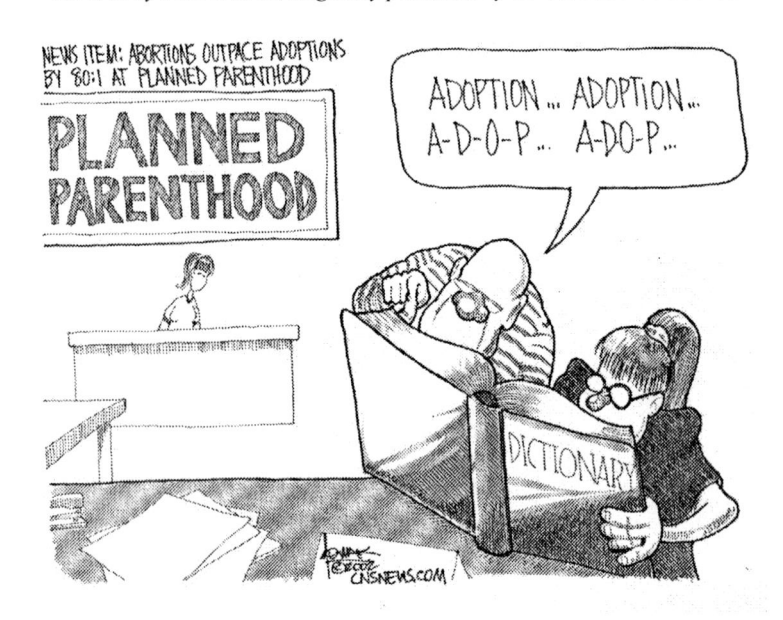

Cartoon by Paul Nowak, originally published by CNSnews.com on 5/9/02

Cartoon by Paul Nowak, originally published by CNSnews.com on 8/31/05

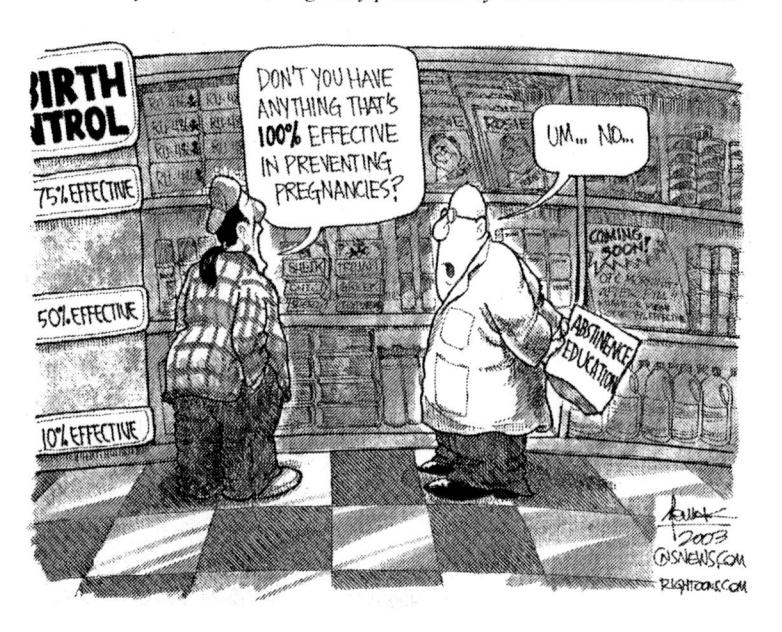

Pro-abortion advocates admit that pregnant women are more likely targets for violent acts – in fact homicide is the leading cause of death in pregnant women. But pro-abortion groups, including Planned Parenthood, oppose laws that would count such violence as crimes against two people. They would rather ignore the emotional pain a woman suffers when her child is taken from her, and impose what they call "enhanced penalties" for harm done to a pregnant women. Why? They fear that recognizing the unborn child as a person could shut down their lucrative business.

Keep an eye on bills or laws that come up dealing with these issues, and you will notice that Planned Parenthood usually sends speakers to testify at hearings, lobby the legislature, and ultimately file lawsuits to block the laws if passed. Pro-life organizations like LifeNews.com continually monitor such actions around the country.

There is an eerie resemblance between such action from the abortion industry and the tobacco industry. Both have tried to offer self-regulation (and protect it) to prevent state or federal limitations, and both have set up research organizations (Alan Guttmacher Institute for Planned Parenthood, and the Council for Tobacco Research and the Tobacco Institute for tobacco companies). Both industries have developed campaigns for young people, supposedly for the purpose of deterring unhealthy activity, and both have been found to have lied and misrepresented health risks to protect their interests. In fact, millions of dollars in research was spent by Big Tobacco to try to downplay or prove that tobacco did not cause cancer, just as pro-abortionists are downplaying the abortion-breast cancer link.

Cartoon by Paul Nowak, originally published by CNSnews.com on 8/31/05

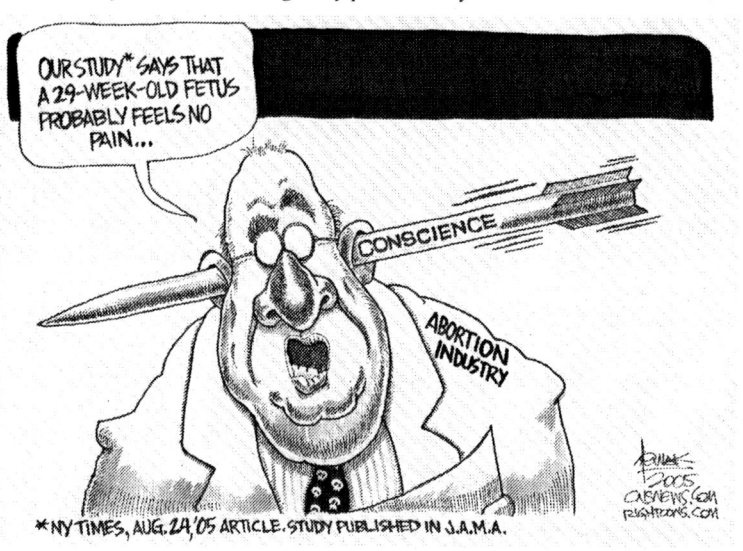

Tobacco companies have also been accused of promoting chewing tobacco as a safe alternative to smoking, while Planned Parenthood is well known for promoting supposedly "safe sex" with birth control devices and pills.

Would anyone trust a tobacco company representative who said smoking was completely safe? Why then do people believe the billion-dollar abortion industry when they say abortion is safe?

Question 8: What did the leaders of the early feminist movement think about abortion?

Abortion advocacy has become synonymous with the modern feminist movement. Groups such as the National Organization for Women (NOW) have become so outspoken in their abortion rights campaign that the group is seen as "pro-abortion" as much or more than it is seen as "feminist." In fact, one of the most recognized feminist groups today that is not pro-abortion has to specify that fact in its name: Feminists for Life.

This was not always the case. Early pioneers for women's rights did not ignore the issue of abortion, even though it was illegal at the time and a taboo subject. In fact, they were outspoken about the matter – but only to criticize the practice, and connect it with the very subjugation of women that they rallied and fought so hard against.

Susan B. Anthony, a leader of the early feminist movement and co-founder of the feminist newspaper "The Revolution," denounced the practice of abortion in the July 8, 1869 edition of her paper, calling it "child-murder."

She added that while the woman who aborts her child is at fault (a common theme at the time in articles condemning the practice) she identified the greater fault from one who subjugated her to the act:

"Guilty? Yes. No matter what the motive, love of ease, or a desire to save from suffering the unborn innocent, the woman is awfully guilty who commits the deed. It will burden her conscience in life, it will burden her soul in death; But oh, thrice guilty is he who drove her to the desperation which impelled her to the crime!"

Anthony did not believe that a law against abortion was enough; she demanded sought "prevention, not punishment" for she saw abortion as a symptom of a greater oppression of women.

"To my certain knowledge this crime is not confined to those whose love of ease, amusement and fashionable life leads them to desire immunity from the cares of children: but is practiced by those whose inmost souls revolt from the dreadful deed, and in whose hearts the maternal feeling is pure and undying. What, then has driven these women to the desperation necessary to force them to commit such a deed? This question being answered, I believe, we shall have such an insight into the matter as to be able to talk more clearly of a remedy."

The Revolution's other co-founder, Elizabeth Cady Stanton, was equally opposed to abortion. In the March 12, 1868 edition of the paper she also linked it to the disenfranchisement and downtrodden state of women.

"There must be a remedy even for such a crying evil as this. But where shall it be found, at least where [will it] begin, if not in the complete enfranchisement and elevation of women?"

In a letter to Julia Ward Howe in October of 1873, Stanton repeated this sentiment:

"When we consider that women are treated as property, it is degrading to women that we should treat our children as property to be disposed of as we see fit."

These two founding mothers of women's rights were not alone in their belief that abortion exemplified everything they opposed:

"When a man steals to satisfy hunger, we may safely conclude that there is something wrong in society - so when a woman destroys the life of her unborn child, it is an evidence that either by education or circumstances she has been greatly wronged."
-Mattie Brinkerhoff in *The Revolution, September 2, 1869*

"The rights of children as individuals begin while yet they remain the foetus."
-Victoria Woodhull, the first female candidate for U.S. President, in *Woodhull's and Claffin's Weekly, December 24, 1870*

"Every woman knows that if she were free, she would never bear an unwished-for child, nor think of murdering one before its birth."
-Victoria Woodhull in *Wheeling, West Virginia Evening Standard, November 17, 1875*

"Abortion is the ultimate exploitation of women."
 - Alice Paul, author of the original 1923 Equal Rights Amendment (ERA), and opponent of its later inclusion of abortion rights.

"[This] subject lies deeper down in woman's wrongs than any other...I hesitate not to assert that most of [the responsibility for] this crime lies at the door of the male sex."
- Matilda Gage in *The Revolution, April 9, 1868*

"Women becoming, consequently, weaker...than they ought to be...have not sufficient strength to discharge the first duty of a mother; and sacrificing to lasciviousness the parental affection...either destroy the embryo in the womb, or cast it off when born. Nature in every thing demands respect, and those who violate her laws seldom violate them with impunity."
- Mary Wollstonecraft, describing the sexual exploitation of women in her work, *"A Vindication of the Rights of Women"* (1792) reprinted by Susan B. Anthony in *The Revolution.*

"Child murderers practice their profession without let or hindrance, and open infant butcheries unquestioned...Is there no remedy for all this ante-natal child murder?...Perhaps there will come a time when...an unmarried mother will not be despised because of her motherhood...and when the right of the unborn to be born will not be denied or interfered with."
-Sarah Norton, in *Woodhull's and Claffin's Weekly, November 19, 1870*

"The custom of procuring abortions has reached such appalling proportions in America as to be beyond belief...So great is the misery of the working classes that seventeen abortions are committed in every one hundred pregnancies."
Emma Goldman in *Mother Earth, 1911*

Have women really been emancipated? Have they, in fact, come such a long way since the suffragist pioneers? They are able to vote, hold political office, and have made great strides toward obtaining equal pay. They have careers, and the appearance of being peers to men.

Cartoon by Paul Nowak, originally published by CNSnews.com on 3/1/04

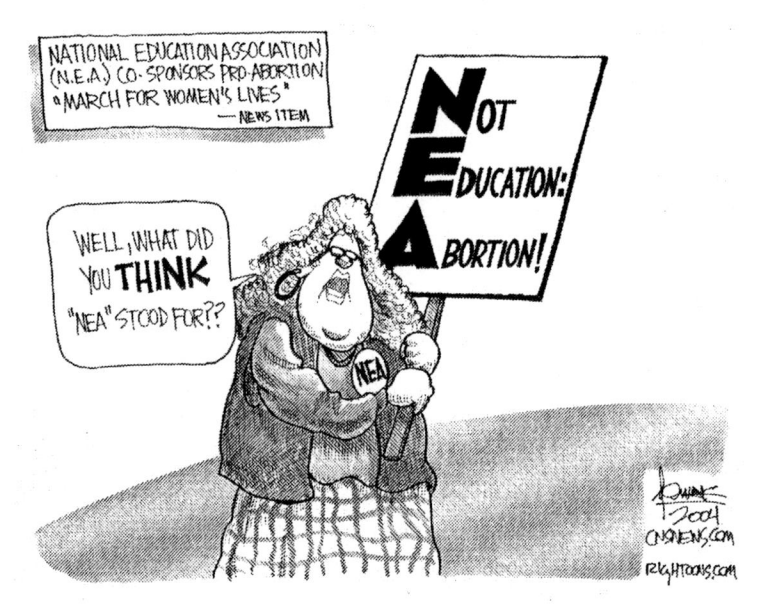

Abortion, however, has been embraced by the daughters of those who so vehemently opposed it. The "modern" feminist movement has resulted in women dressing to please men, and pornography is more readily accessible and more profitable an industry than ever before. Yes, abortion has come out of the actual and figurative "back alley," from being taboo to being a common, and even celebrated practice, but with it has come other forms of the exploitation of women – mainstream pornography, legalized prostitution, and the expectation of sexual promiscuity.

Indeed, the founding mothers of women's rights could not possibly equate the pro-life movement as a backward step to the Dark Ages. It is their heiresses, the daughters of the movement, who have condemned their sisters and daughters to a slavery to men that could not have been conceived by their great-grandmothers.

Viktor Frankl, the Jewish psychiatrist who survived Auschwitz, discussed sexual morality from a psychiatrist's point of view in his book *Man's Search for Ultimate Meaning*. He remarked that, compared to the promiscuity embraced by modern feminists, prostitutes were more praiseworthy:

"As compared with the hypocrisy of businessmen working in the field of so-called sex education, I praise the honesty of the call girls who bluntly confess they are only out to make money through sex ... as to promiscuity, it not only is a type of regressive behavior but also contradicts the humanness of man."

Frankl also writes:

"Thus, promiscuity ... [is the mark] of fixation at, or regression to, immature levels of development. Therefore it is not wise to glorify the indulgence in such patterns of regressive behavior by confusing it with a progressive mentality."

In 1910, the Christian philosopher G.K. Chesterton remarked in his book, *What's Wrong With the World,* that the definition of a Feminist was "one who dislikes the chief feminine characteristics" for so adamantly wishing to be like men. It is my opinion that if the Feminist of Chesterton's time disliked women, the present day feminist must hate her sex so much she is bent on its enslavement and destruction.

Question 9: Is population control a reason to justify abortion?

I once heard Cardinal Francis Arinze, Chairman of Vatican Inter Religious Dialogue, address this very question. He remarked that when you have guests over for dinner and discover that there is not enough food for everyone, the solution is not to kill the guests!

Cardinal Arinze's parable illustrates that using population limits as an excuse for permitting abortion is a nearsighted solution that ignores other, more viable options. Are we certain that there isn't enough food on the table for everyone? Is there really a population problem that requires consideration of so drastic a remedy as abortion?

After years of hype about an impending "population explosion," evidence is mounting that a population implosion in more likely. In 2003, the United Nations Population Division (UNPD) projected the possibility of the world population declining from the current 6.3 billion to 2.3 billion by 2300.

The U.N.'s other predictions of an ever-increasing world population, however, have been more popular in media reports. Such reports have been criticized as being too optimistic by watchdog groups. Researchers at the Population Research Institute pointed out that the UNPD inexplicably assumed in the more "populous" reports that fertility rates would not drop below 1.85 children per woman, despite the fact that in some areas the fertility rate is already below that figure. Italy, for instance, had a fertility rate of only 1.3 in 2003 – a particularly bleak number when a rate of at least 2.1 is necessary to maintain a population's size. In fact, as of 2004, not a single country in the European Union had a fertility rate at or equal to 2.1. Think about it - if every couple only had one child (or every woman), each generation would be half the size of the preceding one!

The toll of shrinking fertility rates is already taking place. Numbers among the older generations are rapidly outpacing the younger generations. Japan, a country expected by the U.N. to lose as much as 20% of its population in the next few decades, has only 14% of its population made up by persons under the age of 15. Reports in Far Eastern countries have been heard about the difficulty for young men to find brides, as families have fewer children, and, having a cultural preference for boys, produce fewer female babies. In the United States, Americans have expressed concern over the future of Social Security, a program that is dependent on the younger generation to support the older generations.

Even if the world's population is growing, we are certainly not running out of room. If the entire world's population of 6 billion lived in the United States (roughly 3.6 million square miles), the population density would be about 1,600 people per square mile. Since the U.S. Census bureau reported in 2000 that New Jersey had a population density of just over 1,100 people per square mile, the U.S. would be just a little more crowded than New Jersey already is – and the rest of the world would be empty!

By the way, if we all lived like people do in New York City (population density of 26,400 per square mile) we would all fit in an even *smaller* area.

Now that we see how little space humans actually occupy, it is not hard to see that food production could easily meet the world population's need. Unequal distribution of wealth and resources contribute far more to starvation and malnutrition than population growth does.

The U.N.'s designated expert at the U.N. Conference in Rome in 1996 stated that five billion dollars a year, not including distribution costs, would be sufficient to pay for enough food to stop all of the world's malnutrition. This amount is far less than the $39 billion the United States spent on foreign aid in 2004 (according to the Congressional Research Service). Spent properly, a handful of the world's wealthiest nations could afford to end starvation around the world.

Does it really make sense to "shoot the guests" at the world's dinner table? Certainly not – we have enough room and enough food. If we are running short on anything, it appears to be people.

Question 11: Where is the benefit of embryonic stem cell research?

First of all, when the subject of stem cell research comes up, it is important to distinguish the two major types:

1) Adult stem cell research, which uses still-developing cells that can replicate and become other, similar cells. Dozens of cures and treatments for diseases and conditions have been derived from adult stem cells, which are harvested without loss of human life. They can be found, for instance, in umbilical cord blood, or even baby teeth. Since there is no destruction of human life involved, this type of research is embraced by pro-life groups.

2) Embryonic stem cells, which uses stem cells harvested from unborn embryos – also referred to as blastocysts for fetal tissue. This type of stem cell is theoretically believed to be more versatile than adult stem cells, but has yet to show any evidence of being useful. As this type of research destroys the developing embryo, it is opposed by pro-life groups.

Proponents of embryonic stem cell research will seldom differentiate for two reasons. First, it adds the credibility of adult stem cell research to the unproven practice they endorse, and secondly because they claim that opponents of embryonic stem cell research are against both kinds of research.

Perhaps the strongest argument against embryonic stem cell research to use with someone who does not share your views is that public funds should not go to untried and untested theories. No clinical trials have been done on humans, and studies using embryonic stem cells in animals have sometimes resulted in teratomata – large tumors of semi-differentiated cells, sometimes even growing hair and teeth. Indeed, to give public funding to research that has provided more harm than good (as the state of New Jersey has already done) is the equivalent of giving grants to snake-oil salesmen. When you consider the fact that human lives are destroyed in the process, the research becomes inexcusable.

In August 2005, Dr. James Dobson drew a parallel that further explained why embryonic stem cell research should not be conducted, especially with taxpayers' money:

"In World War II, the Nazis experimented on human beings in horrible ways in the concentration camps, and I imagine, if you wanted to take the time to read about it, there would have been some discoveries there that benefited mankind," said Dobson.

Dobson went on to explain that a utilitarian approach, one that considers a method good if the results are good, is an incorrect approach.

"We condemn what the Nazis did because there are some things that we always could do but we haven't done, because science always has to be guided by ethics and by morality. And you remove ethics and morality, and you get what happened in Nazi Germany," said Dobson.

Considering that adult stem cell research has been proven to be effective, why waste time, money, and human lives on research that is of no benefit?

Besides – shouldn't organ donorship be voluntary?

Question 12: How is ending someone's life prematurely showing respect for the elderly or the disabled?

Whenever I hear euthanasia being discussed, I am reminded of a story from Grimm's Fairy Tales:

Once, there was a little old man who lived with his son and his son's wife. He had grown feeble with age, and his hands trembled. Whenever he ate, his trembling hands made the silverware clatter, and he would spill food on himself and the table.

The daughter-in-law got quite fed up and impatient with the old man. She and her husband sat him at a separate table in the corner of the kitchen, and gave him an earthenware bowl and wooden spoon to eat with. Each night the old man ate alone, with trembling hands and misty eyes.

One day his hands shook so much that he dropped his bowl and it broke. His son and his daughter-in-law scorned him for his clumsiness and made him use a wooden bowl.

The couple's little son, seeing his grandfather sit in the corner with his wooden bowl, and his parents sitting at the finely set table, watched the grown-ups intently. He then began to gather his blocks, and arrange them on the floor.

"What are you doing, my son?" asked his father.

"I am building a trough," said the child, smiling, "from which to feed my dear parents when they are old."

Cartoon by Paul Nowak, originally published by CNSnews.com on 10/28/03

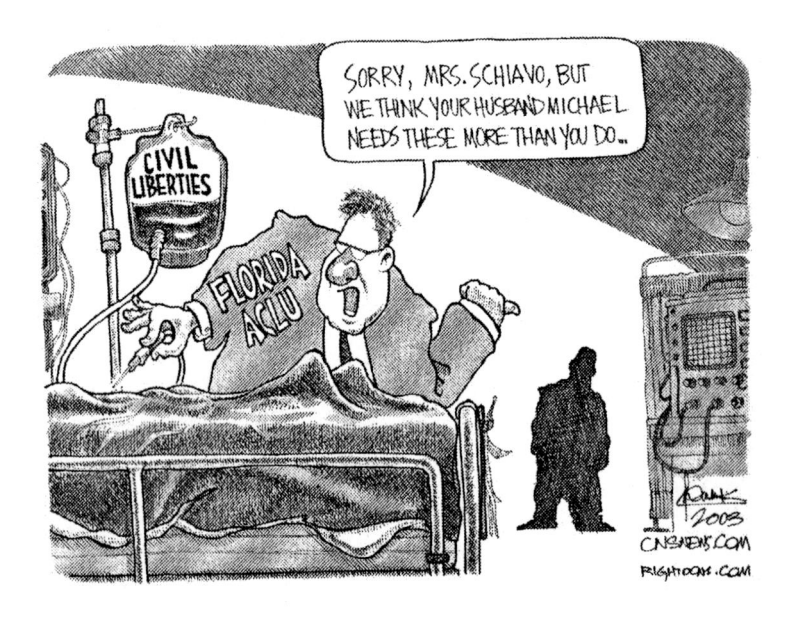

The younger generation is always watching, learning from their parents and elders. Such an idea should be remembered most by lawmakers, parents, and proponents of "mercy killing." The easier one generation makes it to legally hasten the death of the elderly, the more certainly they themselves will one day have their lives placed in the hands of a child, health care worker, or insurance company employee who once sat assembling a trough, learning from their elders how to treat the aging.

The "slippery slope" that has been mentioned in many pro-life articles on the subject is no longer a warning or a fear; evidence of "mercy killings" being performed on the elderly without their full consent is growing.

- In 2002, the president of the Vermont Medical Society, Dr. Lloyd Thompson, ended the life of an 85-year-old patient without her consent or that of her family. Following an investigation by the Attorney General and the state Medical Practice Board, Dr. Thompson only received a reprimand for his actions, and was allowed to continue practicing without interruption.

- In the wake of hurricane Katrina in 2005, there were reports of medical personnel "ending the suffering" of dozens of critically ill patients in area hospitals.

- In 2002, an Oregon doctor who supported assisted suicide, Dr. Peter Rasmussen, told an audience of supporters in Vermont that if a patient did not die from the standard dose of barbiturate tablets, they were given a liquid dose. This testimony raised alarms among concerned doctors, as no ingestible barbiturate existed – only an injectable drug, used to put animals down. If doctors in Oregon were actually using this liquid barbiturate, pentobarbital, they would have to be injecting their patients with it, actively ending their lives in violation of Oregon's law.

- In 2001, Michael Freeland of Oregon was given a prescription for a lethal dose of medication in order to end his life, even though he was not terminally ill, or, according to the doctor who gave him the prescription, capable of making serious medical decisions for himself due to depression. Both mental competency and terminal illness are requirements for legal assisted suicide under Oregon law.

- The highly publicized case of Terri Schiavo, who died of starvation in March of 2005, highlighted the plight of those who are incapable of making decisions for themselves. Ultimately, as in Terri's case, these peoples' lives are ultimately in the hands of others, who can be given the legal power to kill them.

The approval of suicide, assisted suicide, and euthanasia of the disabled, mentally handicapped, and elderly makes a statement that they are no longer considered a benefit to society. By classifying them as groups that are disposable, their dignity, our respect for them, and the contributions they are still able to make to the human race, are lost forever.

Question 13: Is the death penalty really a deterrent to crime? If so, why isn't it working?

The death penalty is not usually a topic covered in pro-life discussions. I include it here because it should be considered by those who use the title "pro-life." If there is any reason to justify the premature ending of a human life, it potentially opens the door to the ending of any other human life.

The typical defense of the death penalty is that it is a deterrent for crime. However, it is impossible to prove that it is or is not working; all we can know is that crimes are still being committed for which persons have already been executed.

If an execution is being carried out to prevent the person from committing a crime again, how do we know that they would have committed a crime again? Are we not therefore punishing them for something they have not yet done?

If the execution is meant to deter others from committing the same acts as the one being executed, why is the execution done in secret, with only a handful of onlookers? An example must be made in the open, not in secret. After all, the crime itself is often done in secret. Consider also that the onlookers, if there are any, are usually related to the person the crime was committed against. They, I am sure, are not likely to repeat a crime that has hurt them so greatly. However, since they alone are permitted to watch, it makes the entire act appear very much to be that of revenge.

In his 1957 essay *Reflections on the Guillotine,* Algerian philosopher Albert Camus noted that even when executions were public, they did not deter criminal activity in others. Statistics from the early 1900s show that of 250 persons that were hanged, 170 had attended one or more executions, and of 167 men that were executed at a Bristol prison in 1886, 164 had witnessed an execution. Yet we cannot prove how many, if any, people have not committed a crime because they feared the death penalty.

Another question that should be asked is whether or not death is really a just and fair punishment – after all, everyone dies whether they commit a heinous crime or not. If one is religious, of course, execution may be seen as expediting a person's day of judgment – but then is salvation and a chance to make amends denied because an executioner chose the time of death, and not God? If one does not believe in God, death is even less of a punishment. The executed is freed from life and sent to the void, where he cannot suffer or know pain. Would it not be more painful to keep them alive, cut off from society and the rights and happiness freedom offers? Let them stop living among humans and know they are missing something, instead of ending their consciousness, leaving the victims' families to be the only ones to suffer the consequences of the crime.

Finally, the argument that is most often made against the death penalty nowadays is the probability of human error, and the growing number of those who have been exonerated before execution by last minute evidence. Once the sentence of death is carried out, it cannot be reversed. Reparations can be made to the imprisoned, and freedom restored. However, what Camus wrote in 1957 is still true today in the 21st Century: "The science that claims to prove innocence as well as guilt has not yet reached the point of resuscitating those it kills."

Question 14: What if you're wrong?

This final conscience prick can be the most powerful question you can ask, and most often you may never know its result.

We all doubt our beliefs and perceptions at some point, and by asking this you could cause a pro-abortion opponent to reconsider their position. Probably not immediately, but maybe a few hours, days, weeks or even years later they may wonder, "What if I *am* wrong?"

You cannot change someone's mind, you have to let them change it. You can point out the facts and the truth of the matter, but unless they convince themselves they are wrong, they are not going to change their beliefs or position.

There is evidence that many may already be unsure of where they stand on the abortion issue. They may simply respond to polls that they are "pro-choice" because its the politically correct response, without really thinking it through.

A June 2003 poll of Democratic caucus-goers in Iowa, funded by the Planned Parenthood Action Fund and the Freedom Fund of Planned Parenthood of Greater Iowa, found that 66% percent of the members of the predominately pro-abortion party considered themselves "pro-choice," but 63% percent did not agree with Planned Parenthood or their party leaders that abortion should be legal and generally available without restriction.

I myself witnessed the pro-choice identity crisis in high school. A student came to my table at lunch one day and asked if anyone was pro-life. I said I was. She was relieved, for she had asked at every table and could not find anyone who said they were pro-life. She had to argue the pro-life cause against abortion in a debate class, but being pro-choice herself she didn't know what points to make.

I asked her what her own views were on abortion. "Only if the mother and baby can't survive," she replied, mentioning ectopic pregnancies which, in addition to being lethal for the baby, can be extremely dangerous and often fatal for the mother. I told her that her position was far closer to being pro-life than pro-choice. When we met later to review her materials for the debate the next day, she had already put together a strong case from her own research and beliefs.

She later told me she won the debate, hands down. Her opponent, another "pro-choice" student, could hardly defend her own position, much less make a case for her beliefs.

Since then I have met several people who initially tell me they are "pro-choice," but as we discuss the issue further their beliefs turn out to be more in line with the pro-life position than that of Planned Parenthood and other pro-abortion groups.

So when closing a discussion of life issues, whether your opponent is stunned and needs time to think things over, or is resolute that their position is right, ask them, "What if you are wrong?" and let them convince themselves.

Recommended Resources

To find more information to help you defend life, the following resources are suggested:

LifeNews.com
Pro-life news service covering all facets of the pro-life movement.

Elliott Institute – www.afterabortion.org
An organization that monitors and compiles research on abortion's effects on the physical and psychological health of women.

National Right to Life Committee – www.nrlc.org
The nation's largest pro-life organization.

American Life League – www.all.org
Another national pro-life organization that provides numerous outreach programs, among them STOPP, which is dedicated to curbing Planned Parenthood's agenda.

The Susan B. Anthony List – www.sba-list.org
Pro-life organization that focuses on political action, providing support for pro-life women in government and providing training for campaign staff and grassroots activists.

The Population Resource Institute – www.POP.org
PRI is dedicated to dispelling the myth of overpopulation and ending abuses of human rights around the world committed in the name of family planning.

NOTES

The art of apologetics requires a persistent willingness to learn and grow. Use the following pages to write down questions for which you need to look up answers, arguments or statistics that support the pro-life position, or other pieces of information helpful for explaining your position.

NOTES

About the Author

Paul E. Nowak is the author of *Guerrilla Apologetics for Catholics*, and owns and operates R.A.G.E. Media. His writing credits include freelance reporting for LifeNews.com, public relations work for Franciscan University of Steubenville, and freelance articles for various publications including the *Philadelphia Inquirer* and CatholicExchange.com.

Paul lives in New Jersey with his wife, Jennifer, and their three children.

About the Illustrator

Paul A. Nowak is a freelance illustrator, whose political cartoons regularly appear on CNSnews.com, Rightoons.com, and in newspapers around the country (when they have the courage or lack of judgment to print his work). A veteran of the U.S. Coast Guard, the U.S. Naval Reserve, and the U.S. Marine Corps, Paul has been drawing cartoons since 1993 when he drew a weekly comic strip for a newspaper in Japan.

Paul resides in Chicago in a converted refrigerator box under an overpass.

The author and illustrator are not related (or at least are not aware of any familial ties).

Guerrilla Apologetics
To order more copies of this book, or for information about other products, visit **www.GApologetics.com** or write:

**Paul Nowak
PO Box 401
Mt. Laurel, NJ 08054**

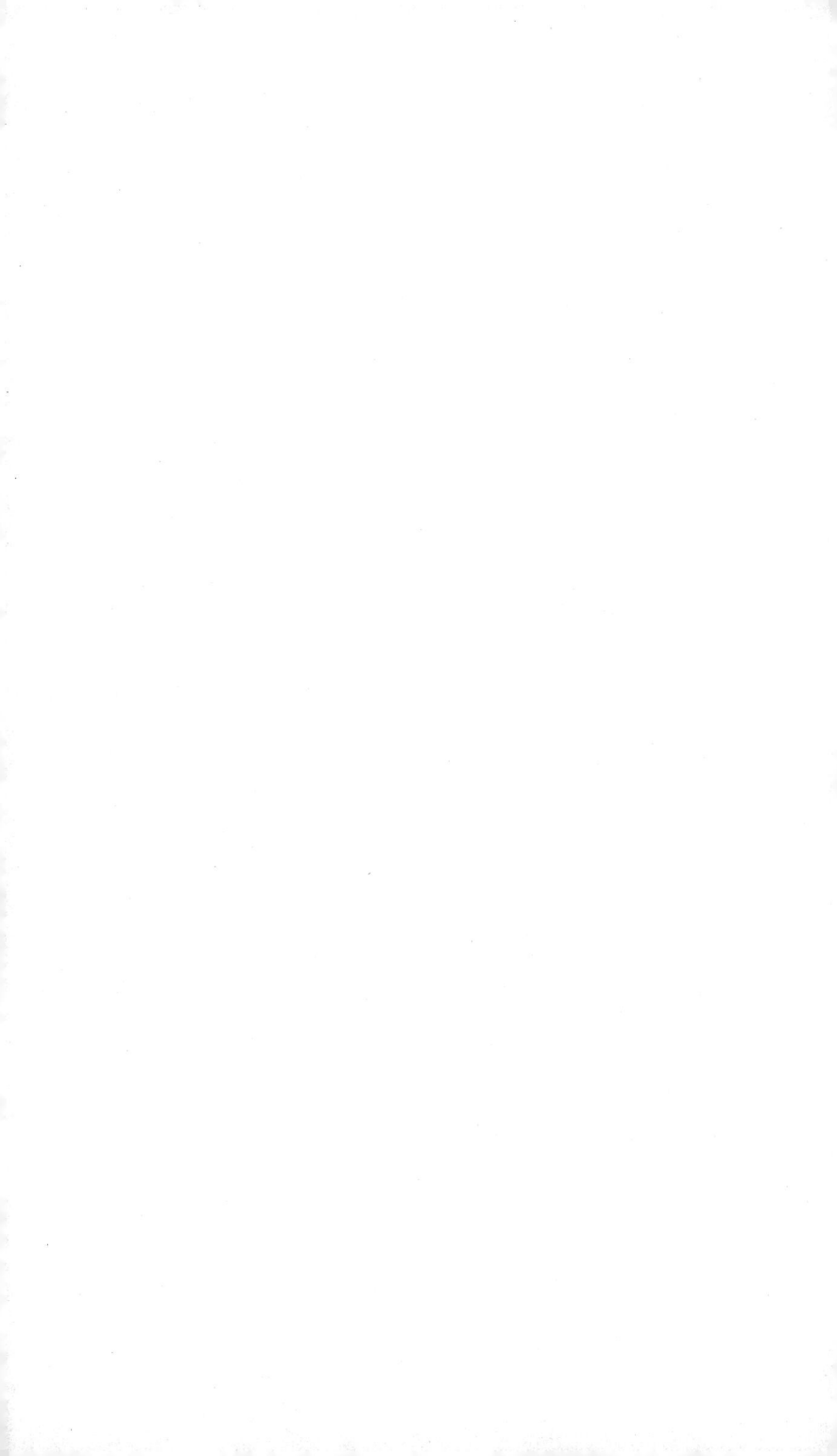

Printed in the United States
40036LVS00001B/136-162